ALYSON MCWILLIAMS

Sacred Beginnings, Healing Endings.

Inspirations to Open and Close Your Yoga Practice

To my mother, who saw what I couldn't see who knew what I needed before I did. Thank you for taking me on my first yoga retreat when my life was filled with the stress and demands of a corporate job. It was your intuition, love and guidance that led me to a path of healing and transformation. Because of you, yoga found me at a time when I needed it the most, and it changed the course of my life. Your support and belief in me lit the way to a journey of self-discovery, peace, and purpose.

Contents

Introduction

Welcome to Sacred Beginnings, Peaceful Endings: Inspirations to Open and Close Your Yoga Practice.

Over the past 15+ years of owning and operating my yoga studio, I've had the honor of guiding countless students on their yoga journeys. For the past six years, I've also led our 200-hour Yoga Teacher Training, witnessing firsthand the transformative power of this practice not only for students but for the teachers stepping into their roles as guides and mentors.

One of the most common challenges I hear from both new and experienced teachers is the struggle to find the right words. Whether it's setting the tone at the start of class or offering a closing sentiment to leave students with a sense of peace and fulfillment, many teachers feel unsure about what to say. This book was born to address that need.

In Sacred Beginnings, Peaceful Endings, you'll discover a thoughtfully curated collection of inspirational words and phrases designed to help you open and close your yoga classes. These mantras and reflections are more than words they are tools to create a sacred space, connect with your students on a deeper level, and leave a lasting impression that extends well beyond the mat.

Each section of the book offers different ways to inspire and support your teaching:

- Opening: Use these passages at the start of your class, when students have settled onto their mats whether in child's pose, easy seat, or any pose that grounds them into the present moment.
- Little Nuggets: These are brief insights to be shared while students are holding poses, offering moments of introspection and inspiration to deepen their practice.
- Closing: Share these closing passages as your students rest in Savasana, allowing them to absorb the practice fully and leave with a sense of calm and completion.

Additionally, the final chapter is devoted to themed openings and closings for special days and holidays, giving you meaningful words for every occasion.

My hope is that this book will not only ease the anxiety of "not knowing what to say," but also inspire you to discover and embrace your own unique voice as a teacher. As you explore these pages, remember that your words carry power they can uplift, motivate, and heal. May this book help you create a space where your students feel seen, heard, and inspired.

The Light in Me Honors the Light in You,

Alyson

And Now The Practice Of Yoga

Opening: Arrive as You Are: A Warm Welcome to Your Practice

Welcome… In whatever way you're showing up here… wherever you may have been… Gather your whole self up and let yourself know you are welcome here… Whether you're showing up with expectations, fears, joy, or sorrow… Take a moment to greet yourself exactly as you are right now… Gather yourself up and welcome all of you. Your mind, your body, and your breath… From this place, create your intention.

Closing: As we come to the end of our practice, take a moment to honor the space you've created for yourself today. You've welcomed all parts of who you are your mind, body, and breath just as they are. Carry this sense of acceptance and presence with you as you step off your mat, knowing that you are whole, exactly as you are. Let your intention continue to guide you, not just here, but in all that you do. Take one last deep breath, and as you exhale, feel the connection to yourself and to this moment.

Opening:"Breath Before Movement: Building a Connection to Your Practice"

Before you create a relationship with your practice, let's first establish a deep connection to your breath. The breath is the bridge between your body and mind, anchoring you in the present moment. Let's begin with mindful breathing Inhale deeply to a count of 1, 2, 3, 4… hold for just a moment, feeling the fullness of that breath. Now, gently exhale for 4, 3, 2, 1, releasing any lingering tension or thoughts. Feel how each breath nourishes your body and creates space within. With every inhale, invite in a feeling of calm, clarity, and openness. With every exhale, let go of what no longer serves you whether it's physical tightness, mental clutter, or emotional weight.

Continue this rhythmic breathing, allowing it to guide you into a state of balance and peace. Let this relationship with your breath lay the foundation for your practice today, grounding you in presence and inviting you to move with intention and ease.

Closing: As we close our practice, return once more to the breath that guided you. Inhale deeply for 1, 2, 3, 4… hold for a moment, feeling that sense of fullness, and gently exhale for 4, 3, 2, 1. Notice the calm that has settled within you, the connection you've nurtured between your mind, body, and breath. Take this moment to honor the journey you've been on today the space you've created, the energy you've released, and the peace you've cultivated. Remember that this breath, this sense of calm and presence, is always with you, ready to support you beyond the mat. As you inhale, gather in the strength, clarity, and balance from your practice. And as you exhale, let go of any remaining tension, allowing yourself to feel light and centered. Carry this connection with you throughout your day, remembering that in every moment, you can return to your breath. The breath is your anchor, your guide, and your constant source of inner peace. Take one last deep breath in, hold it gently, and with a slow, peaceful exhale, release into the present.

Opening: "Listening Inward: A Meditation to Find Stillness and Self-Care"

Meditation is simply listening listening deeply to the whispers of your body, the rhythm of your breath, and the stillness within. Remember, I have nothing to give anybody if I don't first give to myself. So, give yourself permission to step away from the noise, the busyness, and the demands of life. Step into this sacred space where you can truly listen. Listen to your body, the sensations it's offering you. Listen to your breath, its natural ebb and flow, and allow it to guide you home to yourself. At this moment, there's nothing you need to change, nothing you need to fix. Simply be, and let yourself rest in the knowing that *all is well, all is well.*

As you continue to listen, trust that whatever arises is exactly what you need to hear. Whether it's peace or discomfort, joy or stillness, embrace it all with compassion. You are exactly where you need to be. Take this sense of deep listening with you as you leave your mat, carrying the inner peace and wisdom you've cultivated today. No matter what lies ahead, return to this breath, this body, and this truth: *all is well.*

Little Nugget: When you find stillness, see if you can explore more softness. Soften the jaw, the shoulders, even the mind.

Closing: As we bring our practice to a close, let's take a moment to honor the simple act of listening to your body, to your breath, and to the stillness within. Throughout this practice, you've given yourself the gift of presence, of tuning into your own needs, and allowing whatever arises to simply be. Just as we stepped into this space to listen deeply, carry that sense of mindful listening with you off the mat. In the midst of the busyness of life, remember that you always have permission to step away, to pause, to reconnect.

Trust that in each moment, regardless of circumstances, there is a place within you that is steady and whole. As you take one last breath together, inhale deeply, feeling the fullness of the present, and exhale softly, letting go of anything you no longer need. And know that, wherever you go, you can return to this truth: *all is well, all is well.*

Opening:"Namaste: A Salutation of Connection and Self-Respect"

Namaste is both a salutation and a way to show your connection to those around you. It is also a sign of respect towards yourself and all beings around you
　I see what is holy in you
　I see what is noble in you
　I see what is beautiful in you
　I love and respect you without conditions
　The light in you shines bright

Closing: As we come to the end of our practice, let's take a moment to honor the meaning of *Namaste is* a recognition of our shared connection, a deep respect for ourselves and for each other. I see what is holy in you. I see what is noble and beautiful in you. I love and respect you without conditions, and I honor the light that shines so brightly within you. May this light guide you through your day and remind you of the beauty in yourself and all beings around you.

Opening: "Anchored in Breath: Coming Home to Yourself"

As you come to your mat, gently close your eyes and focus on your breath. Feel the natural rhythm of the inhale and exhale. Each breath is an invitation to come home to yourself. Let the breath be your anchor, grounding you in the now, where all things begin.

Closing: As we close our practice, return to your breath your steady anchor throughout our time together. Notice its gentle rhythm, the rise and fall, and how it brings you back home to yourself. Remember that this breath is always available to you, a constant invitation to ground yourself in the present moment. As you move forward from your mat and into your day, carry this sense of calm and centeredness with you. Let your breath guide you back whenever you need to find stillness, whenever you need to reconnect with yourself.

Opening: Cultivating Gratitude

Before we begin our practice today, let's take a moment to cultivate gratitude. Think of one thing no matter how small that you're thankful for right now. Hold it in your heart as you move through this practice, and let it be your guide. When we lead with gratitude, the world becomes a little brighter.

Closing: As we close our practice, let gratitude continue to guide you. Remember that even the smallest moments of thankfulness can bring light to your day. Carry this feeling in your heart, letting it shape your thoughts, your actions, and the way you see the world around you. When we move with gratitude, we open ourselves to endless possibilities of joy and connection

Opening: "From Thinking to Feeling: A Practice of Release and Presence"

Take a moment to move from thinking to feeling. Feel into the rise and fall of the breath, letting each inhale and exhale become more audible, more present. Allow your awareness to shift from the chatter of the mind to the sensations within your body the gentle expansion of the ribs as you breathe in, the grounding sensation as you breathe out.

From this place of feeling and awareness, ask yourself, *'What can I let go of that has been weighing on me?'* Whether it's a thought, an expectation, an emotion, or an energy, give yourself permission to set it aside just for the next 45, 60, or 90 minutes. Imagine that with each exhale, you are releasing that weight, making space for ease and clarity. Let the breath cleanse you, creating an open space for whatever arises in your practice today. Embrace the possibility that for this time, you are free to simply be, exactly as you are

Little Nugget: Challenge yourself to stay for one more breath…
then one more… and notice how capable you are.

Closing: As we close our practice, take a moment to return to
that intention of letting go of releasing what has been weighing
on you. Notice how the simple act of focusing on your breath
and moving with awareness has created space within you space
to breathe, space to feel, and space to just *be*. Allow yourself to
sit with this sense of freedom, however it may show up for you
right now. And know that even though our practice on the mat
is coming to an end, the choice to let go, to create space, and
to come back to your breath is always available to you. Take a
deep breath in, filling yourself with all the energy, clarity, and
peace from this practice. And as you exhale, let go of anything
you no longer need, knowing that you are lighter, freer, and
more connected to yourself than when you began. Carry this
sense of lightness and openness with you as you leave the mat,
and remember that each breath is an invitation to let go and to
return to the present.

**Opening: You are what your deepest desire is. As your
desire is, so is your intention. As your intention is, so is
your deed. As your deed is, so is your destiny." - *Upanishads***

As we step onto our mats today, let's reflect on these powerful
words. They remind us that everything starts from within
our desires, our intentions, and our actions shape the path of
our lives. So, I invite you to take a moment to turn inward
and connect with your deepest desire. What do you want
to cultivate in your life? It might be peace, strength, self-
compassion, or simply the ability to be present. Let this desire

flow into an intention for your practice today. And as we move together, let every breath, every movement, and every moment of stillness be guided by this intention. Know that in this practice, you are not just moving your body you are setting in motion the energy that will carry you toward your destiny. So, let your desire be a guiding light, your intention be the steady flame, and let the actions of this practice today be the spark that ignites transformation. Let's take a deep breath together, and as you exhale, step fully into your practice, knowing that everything you do on the mat echoes beyond it.

Little Nugget: In each pose, there is space to relax. See if you can find that space now, even as you hold strength.

Closing: As we close our practice, return once more to the intention you set at the beginning of our time together the desire that called you to your mat today. Notice how, through each breath, movement, and moment of stillness, you have nurtured this intention, allowing it to take shape within you.

Remember that the work we do on our mats is a reflection of the work we do in our lives. Your deepest desire, your intention, has begun to manifest not only in this practice but in the way you move through the world. As you take your final few breaths here, feel how your intention has woven through every pose, every inhale, and every exhale. Let it ground you, guide you, and continue to inspire your actions long after you leave your mat. Know that as you step into the rest of your day, your intention carries forward, shaping your deeds, and in turn, your destiny. Take a deep breath in, gathering all the energy, clarity, and strength from this practice, and exhale slowly, letting that intention settle deep within. Carry this wisdom with you, trusting that as your desire is, so will be your life.

Opening: "Listening Inward: Finding Presence Through Breath and Awareness"(Students are in Supta Baddha Konasana)

Yoga begins with listening. When we listen, we are giving space to what is. Place one hand onto your heart and one hand onto your belly. Breathe into the hand on your belly, feeling the breath expand from within. Allow yourself to sit in this space, simply noticing the gentle rise and fall of your belly, feeling the weight of the inner thighs grounding you, relaxing the legs down even more. From this place of stillness and awareness, ask yourself, *'What brought you to your mat today?'* Whatever it is whether it's peace, strength, healing, curiosity, or simply a need for space acknowledge it fully. There is no right or wrong answer; just listen to what arises without judgment.

Allow that reason to be held in the breath, filling your belly as you inhale, and softening with each exhale. Feel the connection between your breath, your body, and your intention. Know that whatever brought you here is enough, and it's what will guide you through your practice today. As you move, let that intention be like an anchor, gently pulling you back whenever your mind wanders or your body feels challenged. And remember, just like the breath that flows in and out, you can always come back to this question, this listening, and this space of simply *being*. Let your practice unfold from this place of deep presence and acceptance

Little Nugget: Your experience of the asana changes when you allow the mind to listen to your body rather than letting the mind dictate what you should do or feel. When you let go of expectations and truly listen, the body naturally guides you to where you need to be, creating a deeper, more authentic practice. It's in listening where growth happens—not by forcing, but by allowing.

Closing: As we close our practice, take a moment to honor the way you've listened to your body today, allowing it to guide you rather than pushing or forcing. Notice how this creates a sense of ease, a more honest connection to each pose. Let this practice of listening continue to guide you beyond the mat, trusting that when you tune in, you are exactly where you need to be. With that deep sense of awareness and gratitude, take one final breath together inhale fully, exhale completely, and carry this sense of listening into your day.

Opening: "A Gentle Journey: Embracing Kindness and Awareness in Your Practice"

Set a gentle intention of being kind and receptive toward your unfolding experience. As we move through our practice, know that it is inevitable for your attention to wander—to explore other sensations, sounds, thoughts, and feelings. The idea is not to judge or force yourself back to stillness, but simply to become aware. When you notice your mind drifting, gently guide it back to the breath, back to the body, back to the present moment. Embrace each distraction as part of the journey, treating every sensation and thought with kindness and curiosity. Remember, it's not about staying perfectly focused it's about practicing acceptance of whatever arises, and coming back with a gentle, open heart.

Little Nugget: Soften the space between your eyebrows and release any tension in your jaw.

Closing: Someone once told me to live for the little things in life …

Live for the sunrise and sunset... Where you'll see colors in the sky that usually don't belong.. Live for road trips with the kids... The music you hate but they love…..The embarrassing moment we cast on them that will be shared at dinner's to come.. To live life and not let the fear of failing stop you from living.. Live for the people that surround you with hope, joy and encouragement that remind you the world is not cold or a harsh place.. Live for the little things they will make you realize that this is what life is about , this is what it means to be alive.. Breathe in hold.. Breathe out. …

Opening: It only takes a reminder to breathe

"It only takes a reminder to breathe, a moment to be still, and just like that, something in me settles, softens, make space for imperfection. The harsh voice of judgment drops to a whisper and I remember again that life isn't a relay race; that we will all cross the finish line; that waking up to life is what we were born for. As many times as I forget, catch myself charging forward without even knowing where I'm going, that many times I can make the choice to stop, to breathe, and be, and walk slowly into the mystery"

• Donna Faulds

Closing: As we close our practice today, remember that it only takes a simple reminder to breathe, a single moment to be still, and just like that something within us settles, softens, and makes space for imperfection. When the harsh voice of judgment fades into a whisper, we're reminded that life isn't a race to be won, but a journey to be experienced. No matter how many times we forget and find ourselves rushing through life, we always have the choice to pause, to breathe, and to simply be. So as we leave our mats, carry this gentle awareness with you the permission to slow down, to let go of striving, and to walk slowly into the unfolding mystery of each moment. Take one last deep breath in, filling yourself with presence, and let it go with a soft exhale, knowing that you are exactly where you need to be.

Opening - "Cultivating Compassion: A Practice of Self-Love and Gentle Release"

Welcome to your practice. Today, let's focus on the theme of compassion both for yourself and for others. As you settle in, take a moment to close your eyes and connect with your breath. Let each inhale fill you with warmth and gentleness, and let each exhale be a soft release of any judgment or tension. Compassion starts within. It's about being kind to yourself, embracing all the parts of you the strong, the struggling, the imperfect, and the growing. Let this practice be a space where you can hold yourself gently, letting go of the need to be anything other than who you are right now. As you move through each posture, approach it with an open heart and a willingness to let go of expectations. And remember, the compassion you cultivate here on the mat is something you can carry with you, sharing that same kindness with those around you. So, let's begin this journey together, one breath, one gentle step at a time.

Closing: As we close our practice, take a moment to reflect on the compassion you've cultivated today the gentle kindness towards yourself, the soft acceptance of wherever you are in this moment. Notice how this compassion has flowed through your breath, your movements, and your thoughts, inviting you to be present with an open heart. Know that this practice doesn't end here; the compassion you've nurtured is something you can carry with you beyond the mat, into every breath, every step, and every interaction. When you encounter challenges or moments of self-doubt, remember the warmth and gentleness you've created within. Take one last deep breath in, gathering all the peace and self-kindness from this practice, and with a slow, complete exhale, release any remaining tension, feeling light and at ease. May you continue to meet yourself and others with compassion, always.

Opening: "Trust the Breath: Finding Strength and Surrender in Your Practice"

Breathe in……. Long exhale notice to be upright is to have an open heart. As the heart opens the mind lets go.. Slow breath in, open your mouth and let it go.. Pause 10 breaths. So as you breathe into the felt experience we learn to let go. Before our bodies can open you must first trust that the breath will carry you. The breath will carry you from high plank to low plank.. No need to rush it.. The breath will hold you up in warrior 2 no need to give up. Trust the breath, trust yourself and let go of the possibility of change.

Closing: As you leave here today, trust that today is going to be a good day, trust that your breath will get you through the highs and lows. Trust that no matter what today brings you it is going to be a good day.

Opening: "Body Love"

Notice what touches the earth. The tops of the feet, knees, arms , palms and each finger that touches the earth. In a few moments I am going to be repeating phrases and I ask that you repeat them inwardly.

- I embrace the challenges…
- I focus on effort not outcome or the end results…
- I am at peace with imperfection…
- I know anything is possible…
- I am going to enjoy the journey every minute for the sake of my mind, body and soul..
- And the last one customize to what you need from this practice and your day/or evening.

Closing: As we close our practice, take a moment to notice what is touching the earth once more the tops of your feet, your knees, arms, palms, and each finger rooted into the ground beneath you. Feel that steady connection, and let it anchor you in this present moment.

Reflect on the words you repeated inwardly, allowing their

meaning to settle deeply within. Remember that you have embraced your challenges, honored your effort, found peace in imperfection, and opened yourself to possibility. Carry that sense of acceptance and presence with you, and let the journey be a source of joy for your mind, body, and soul. And whatever phrase or intention you customized to your needs, let it be a guide for you as you move forward whether into your day or your evening. Know that you can return to this space of grounding and affirmation at any time, letting the earth beneath you hold and support you.Take a deep breath in, gather all the strength and peace from your practice, and as you exhale, release fully into this sense of wholeness and ease.

Opening: "Empowered Within: Cultivating Strength Through Body, Breath, and Mind"

Today, we'll use the physical body, breath, and mind to tap into and embody what it truly means to feel empowered from the deepest parts of your being to the outermost edges of your mind. As you settle into your seat, soften your gaze and bring your awareness inward, focusing on cultivating a sense of mental empowerment. Take a deep inhale, and as you do, imagine tracing a line of breath from the tip of your nose up to your forehead. As you exhale, follow that line down from your forehead back to the nose. With each breath, let it become slower, more deliberate, relaxing the shoulders and softening any tension in the brow. Now, begin to visualize what an empowered mind feels like for you. Maybe it's the ability to make difficult but supported decisions, knowing that the outcome will lead to growth and strength. Whatever empowerment looks like for you, allow yourself to fully feel into that experience each breath fueling and expanding that sense of power within. From this place of inner strength and clarity, let's join together for an OM, letting the sound carry and amplify our intention.

Closing: As we close our practice, take a moment to revisit that sense of empowerment you cultivated within the strength of your breath, the focus of your mind, and the energy of your body all working together. Notice how this feeling has grown and shifted throughout our time together, expanding into every corner of your being. Allow yourself to carry this empowered mindset off the mat knowing that the strength and clarity you've cultivated here is always available to you. Remember, empowerment isn't just about grand gestures; it's about making choices that honor your truth, your growth, and your well-being, even in the small moments.

Opening: "Align & Transform: Finding Your Center Through Yoga"

Take a moment to check in with yourself tune into your body, notice how you're feeling, and acknowledge what you're bringing into this space today. Yoga is a powerful opportunity to step away from the mundane and connect with something deeper, aligning the mind and body to create a sacred experience. It allows us to participate as a community in something transformative. As we begin, I invite you to center yourself and willingly recognize any tension or stress you may be holding. Make a commitment to surrender that tension, allowing yourself to become more present, more open to what unfolds in the next 75 minutes. This practice has the power to change how we relate and react to ourselves and others, so that when we leave this room, we do so with greater openness, awareness, and compassion. Allow your practice to be a space where you release what you no longer need and open your heart to all that awaits.

Closing: As we close our practice, take a moment to reflect on how you feel now having released tension, created space, and reconnected with yourself. Honor the work you've done, not only on a physical level but also on a deeper, more transformative level that extends beyond your mat. Remember that this time has been more than just movement; it's been an opportunity to cultivate openness, presence, and connection. Carry this sense of peace and centeredness with you as you step back into your day, knowing that the awareness you've cultivated here can transform how you show up in your relationships and in the world. Take one last deep breath in, letting it fill you with gratitude and lightness, and a slow, gentle breath out, allowing that sense of calm and openness to stay with you as you move forward.

Opening: "Svadhyaya: The Journey of Self-Study and Inner Reflection"

The term Svadhyaya literally means 'one's own reading' or 'self-study'. It is the fourth Niyama of Patanjali's Yoga Sutras And has the potential to deepen our yoga practice way beyond the mat. It is also one of the three ways to find the state of yoga. To make the unconscious conscious. Through self observation we come to know ourselves. We find the thoughts and feelings that lie behind our actions. We start to see our motivations, it is the process that allows us to change and grow.. In the beginning of my practice I was filled with ego, pushing myself, being hard on myself and even jealous of others who could do more than me. I began to see how these patterns on my mat was how I saw myself in relation to the world. Svadhyaya allows us to observe all our thoughts and emotions whether negative or positive, without judgment and it is in this space that we grow. So I invite you to notice what comes up for you on your mat today without judgment, just pure curiosity.

Closing: As we close our practice, let's honor the journey of *Svadhyaya*—the practice of self-study, reflection, and growth. Today, you took the time to observe yourself honestly, without judgment, and in doing so, you created space to see not just what happens on the mat, but how it reflects your life beyond it. Remember that this process of observing your thoughts and emotions with curiosity, rather than criticism, is where real transformation begins. By bringing awareness to what arises, you create the opportunity to change, grow, and deepen your connection to yourself. As you step off your mat, carry this gentle self-awareness with you. Allow it to guide your interactions, your decisions, and your relationship with yourself, knowing that this practice is always available to help you grow more aligned and present. Take one last deep breath in, honoring the courage to know yourself more fully, and a slow breath out, releasing into a sense of peace and acceptance.

Opening: "Release & Renew: Embracing Heart-Openers and Self-Compassion

I invite you to drop what was never meant for you to hold.

Place one hand on your heart chakra and the other on your belly. Today, my intention is to guide you toward heart openers and to inspire a conversation within yourself around love, forgiveness, compassion, and where you stand in the world today. It's easy to move through life with guilt, anger, hate, entitlement, or denial, forgetting the relationships we create with one another. But at the end of the day, nothing truly matters more than our ability to love and be loved. This is a question I ask myself every day: How will I love today? Not just my kids, friends, or partner, but the world. How am I showing up? And now, my question for you is how will you love today? Take a deep breath into your heart space... and let it go...

Closing: As we come to the close of our practice, take a moment to reflect on the intention set at the beginning to open your heart to love, forgiveness, and compassion. Notice how you feel now, having released what you were never meant to carry. Feel the spaciousness in your heart, the lightness in your breath, and the softness in your spirit. Remember that love is not just a feeling but an action, a choice you can make every day toward yourself, toward others, and toward the world. Carry this openness with you as you leave your mat today. Let it guide your actions, your words, and your thoughts. Ask yourself, 'How will I love today?' and allow the answer to flow through everything you do. Take a deep breath into your heart, honoring all that you are, and exhale, sending that love out into the world.

Opening: "A Dance with Self: Finding Balance and Connection Within"

The power of the heart is to be connected with who you are

at the deepest level. We are in a relationship to center, a relationship for balance. The root meaning of balance is dance. We dance with self, there is a place in our lives for tears, a place in our lives for our grief and while those exist we can look inwardly to the place that lifts us back up. This is part of the practice part of the dance bring that nurturing now back to the self. Breathe into the heart space.

Little Nugget: Notice how your body feels in this pose, and honor it. Self-love is about accepting every sensation, every tight spot, every moment of ease.

Closing: As we close our practice, breathe deeply into your heart space. Remember that the dance of balance is a journey moving gracefully between joy and grief, strength and softness. Embrace all that you are, honoring the tears and the triumphs, knowing they are part of what makes you whole. Let this breath be a nurturing reminder to always come back to your center, back to the heart, where the dance of life continues to lift you up.

Opening: "Always available" - Rosa Park

Rosa Parks once said, "Only when people made up their minds that they wanted to be free and took action was there change." Her words remind us of the incredible power of decision and commitment in creating transformation.

Today, as you step onto your mat, recognize the profound choice you've made to nurture your mind, body, and spirit. This decision is not just a routine it's a powerful action toward your own freedom and growth. Each time you commit to your practice, you're not only taking care of yourself but also becoming a new person, more in tune with who you truly are. As we flow through today's class, feel the strength in your decision. With every pose, with every breath, you are redefining yourself." You are embracing change, releasing old patterns, and stepping into the freedom of your true self. Remember, your practice is an act of courage and self-love. By showing up today, you've already begun the journey of transformation. Let's honor that commitment together and celebrate the new person you continue to become.

Closing: As we close our practice today, take a moment to honor the decision you made to step onto your mat to nurture your mind, body, and spirit. Rosa Parks reminds us that freedom begins with a choice, and by showing up today, you've taken a powerful step toward your own growth and transformation. Breathe deeply and feel the strength in that choice, knowing that each breath and movement has brought you closer to your true self. Remember that this practice is an act of courage, self-love, and freedom, and you carry that strength within you wherever you go. Take one final deep breath, honoring your commitment to yourself and all that you're becoming.

Opening: "Aim and Release: Finding Strength and Direction Through the Bow and Arrow"

In today's practice, we'll draw inspiration from the symbolism of the bow and arrow, a powerful reminder of strength, direction, and the art of letting go. The bow represents the potential within you, the strength you hold to face life's challenges. The arrow is your focus, your direction forward, aiming at your goals and aspirations. As you pull back on the arrow, feel the tension, the resistance that mirrors the stress and challenges in your life. This tension is a necessary part of the journey, teaching us patience, resilience, and the importance of staying true to our path. But just as important as the pull is the release. When you let go of the arrow, you're not just moving forward you're also releasing what no longer serves you. This act of letting go is powerful, freeing, and essential for progress. The arrow shoots forward, unstoppable, not looking back but moving with purpose towards its target. As we flow through today's practice, embody the bow and arrow. Embrace the tension, then release it with trust and intention. Let go of anything holding you back, and move forward with strength, clarity, and purpose.

Closing: As we close our practice, take a moment to embody the symbolism of the bow and arrow one final time. Feel the strength of the bow within you the resilience and potential to face all of life's challenges. And feel the arrow the focus, the direction, the release. Reflect on the tension you may have felt today, both in body and mind, and recognize how letting go has allowed you to move forward. Just as the arrow shoots toward its target, may you move forward with intention, clarity, and purpose in all that you do. Carry this sense of strength and release with you as you step off the mat, trusting in your own power to aim and let go.

Opening: "Crossing the Threshold: Cultivating Courage on the Mat"

Welcome, everyone. As we begin our practice today, I want to take a moment to focus on the theme of courage. It's been said that it takes courage to cross the starting line, but it takes space to cross the finish line. The very act of stepping onto your mat today is an act of courage. You've chosen to show up for yourself, to commit to your well-being, and to embark on a journey of growth and transformation. Let's start this practice by acknowledging that courage the courage it takes to begin, to face challenges, and to keep moving forward, both on and off the mat. But courage alone isn't enough. To reach our goals, to cross the finish line, we need space. Space to breathe, to reflect, to listen to our bodies, and to honor our needs. Throughout our practice today, I invite you to create that space. Allow yourself to be fully present, to move with intention, and to embrace each moment with openness. As we move through our sequences, remember that this time on your mat is not just about the physical practice; it's a celebration of all the ways you show up in life. You are here, giving your best, and that deserves recognition. So let's begin this practice with courage and create the space we need to flourish. Know that by being here today, you're already doing something extraordinary you're giving nothing but your best.

Closing: As we come to the close of our practice, take a moment to honor the courage that brought you here and the space you've created within. You've not only shown up for yourself but have allowed each breath, each pose, and each moment of stillness to be a celebration of your strength and openness. Remember that the courage to start and the space to continue are gifts you can carry off the mat, into all aspects of your life. When challenges arise, find the courage to face them, and the space to breathe through them, knowing that you have everything you need within you to flourish. Take one last deep, spacious breath in, filling yourself with gratitude for this time, and exhale fully, releasing into a sense of peace and strength.

Opening: "Wholehearted Practice: Embracing All That You Are"

You are invited to a yoga practice that honors the fullness of who you are your light, your shadow, and everything in between. In this class, we'll create a space where you can show up exactly as you are. Bring your strength, your joy, and your energy. But also bring your doubts, your fears, and the parts of yourself that you sometimes keep hidden. All aspects of yourself are welcome here. Without judgment, simply notice what arises on your mat today. Every breath and movement is an opportunity to connect with all parts of who you are embracing your wholeness. Know that whatever you bring into this space is enough. You are enough. Allow this practice to be a container for self-exploration, self-acceptance, and self-love, where you can listen, let go, and find ease in simply being.

Little Nugget: Notice what shows up for you at this moment, without judgment. Whether it's strength or struggle, let it all be welcome.

Closing: As we close our practice today, take a moment to honor the fullness of who you are the strength, the vulnerability, the light, and the shadow. You've shown up just as you are, with all that you carry, and that in itself is a beautiful act of self-acceptance. Take one last deep breath in, filling up with the recognition that every part of you is worthy, and as you exhale, release into a space of compassion for your whole self. Carry this feeling with you, knowing that you can always return to this place of wholeness and presence.

Opening: "Union Within: Building a Deep Relationship with Your Body Through Yoga"

With your own body as your partner. When you're new to a pose or just beginning your yoga journey, it can feel intense, like a fire within you. There may be moments when you question whether to push through or sit with the discomfort, trusting that the sensations will pass. It's in those moments that you feel most alive, sensing a connection to something greater than yourself. Yoga invites us to stand at the edge of our comfort zone the place where pure possibility begins. Every time we peel back a layer of ourselves, we arrive at that same edge, faced with a powerful choice. The question isn't whether we can survive stepping out of our comfort zone, but whether we can thrive if we stay within it. Transformation comes when we resist the urge to retreat into the safe, familiar spaces we've created. Instead, we open ourselves to the unknown, asking: *What is available to me right now, in this body, on this mat, in this moment? What can I let go of to show up fully for myself?* It's in this space of surrender that growth becomes possible. Allowing us to evolve and find our strength both on the mat and in our lives.

Closing: As we close our practice, take a moment to honor the edge you stood at today the place where you chose to step beyond comfort and embrace possibility. Remember, it's in the surrender that transformation begins, and by showing up for yourself on the mat, you've already begun that journey. Carry this openness and strength with you, and know that each step outside your comfort zone is a step toward growth and becoming more of who you are meant to be.

Opening: "Gratitude Within: Embracing Self-Appreciation and Inner Strength"

When was the last time you truly thanked yourself? I mean a deep, heartfelt appreciation that reaches your inner core. Take a moment right now to offer gratitude to yourself. Thank yourself for all the hurdles you've overcome and for the strength and grace with which you've navigated life's challenges. Acknowledge the resilience and courage it took to face those obstacles, and honor the perseverance that has brought you to this point. As you reflect on these emotions, notice how your body feels in this moment. Do you feel strong, happy, and empowered, like a resounding "Hell yes, I am a badass"? Embrace that feeling it's a testament to your journey and your strength.

Closing: As we close our practice today, take a moment to thank yourself not just a casual thanks, but a deep, heartfelt gratitude that reaches your core. Thank yourself for showing up, for overcoming challenges, for the resilience and courage it has taken to come this far. Reflect on the strength, grace, and perseverance that have carried you through life's hurdles, and notice how your body feels in this moment. Let yourself feel strong, happy, and empowered like a full 'Hell yes, I am a badass!' Embrace that feeling, knowing that it is a true testament to your journey and your strength. Carry this gratitude and empowerment with you today as you leave these four walls and step into the world.

Opening: "Present Moment Focus: Finding What Matters Most Right Now"

Find yourself in a comfortable position whether seated in Easy Pose or reclining in Supta Baddha Konasana. Take a deep breath in, noticing the sensations within your body, and as you exhale, allow yourself to let go of any tension or thoughts. Now, take another deep breath, and gently ask yourself, 'What is the most important thing in this moment?' Remember that where your awareness goes, your energy flows. Place your hands over your heart, and breathe deeply into that space. Tune into your heart the center of compassion, empathy, and understanding. If there is any part of your life that feels tender or vulnerable, simply observe it without judgment. Hold it softly, as if cradling it with your awareness. Breathe in deeply… and as you exhale, release it all. Let go of anything weighing you down, and feel the lightness that comes from this release. With your next inhale, welcome in compassion, love, and above all, forgiveness, allowing them to fill your heart and your entire being. OM

Closing: As we come to the close of our practice, take one last moment to connect with your heart. Feel the lightness that has come from letting go and the spaciousness created by your breath. Remember that whatever the most important thing is for you right now, you have the power to hold it gently and with compassion. Carry this sense of awareness, love, and forgiveness with you beyond the mat. Trust that as you move through your day, you can always return to this place grounded, open, and connected to your heart. Take a final deep breath in, filling yourself with gratitude, and exhale fully, letting any remaining tension dissolve into peace.

Opening: "Just for Now: Embracing Stillness and Support"

Find yourself in Supta Baddha Konasana, placing one hand on your heart and the other on your belly. Begin by tuning into your breath. Just for now, allow yourself to sink into stillness, without needing to understand how. Let the weight you've been carrying rest upon the earth, feeling the solid support beneath you. Just for now, let each breath be a wave that revitalizes your entire being. As you exhale, release anything that stands between you and your truth. Embrace the feeling of being boundless and free, as energy flows through your hands and feet, awakening every part of you. Breathe in the possibility of fully embodying who you truly are so alive and vibrant that the world seems newly born around you. Just for now... Notice: Begin to notice the natural rise and fall of your breath. Allow your awareness to sink into your lower belly, feeling the gentle movement of your abdomen. As you breathe, relax your shoulders, and start to feel at home within yourself. Let your awareness expand to include everything touching the earth, the temperature on your skin, and the energy of those around you. Connect with this sense of grounding, and from this place, start to form your intention for your practice.

Close your eyes, gently transitioning to slow, steady breaths in and out through your nose. Acknowledge that this is exactly where you need to be. Let go of whatever came before this moment, wiping the slate clean. When we release the past, life becomes lighter and clearer. Take a deep breath in… and a slow, full breath out. From this space of openness and presence, set your intention for today's practice.

Little Nugget: Let the breath clear the slate, creating space for ease and lightness in your practice.

Closing: As we close our practice, take a moment to return to that sense of stillness and presence you cultivated. Feel the support of the earth beneath you, the rhythm of your breath, and the energy within. Remember that just for now, and always, you have permission to let go, to be boundless, and to embrace exactly who you are. Let your intention stay with you as you move into the rest of your day, knowing that you can always come back to this moment of connection and peace. Take one last deep breath in, and a slow, gentle breath out, letting go of all that no longer serves you.

Opening: "Free Your Practice: Letting Go of Expectations and Embracing the Present"

Release any preconceived notions about how your practice should unfold today. Often, we come to the mat with specific goals or ideas in mind whether it's mastering a pose, achieving a certain level of flexibility, or finding a moment of perfect stillness. While these aspirations can be motivating, they can also create unnecessary pressure and hinder the natural flow of your practice. Instead, embrace the present moment and what it has to offer. Your body, mind, and spirit may feel different each time you step onto your mat, and that's perfectly okay.

By letting go of expectations, you create space for authenticity in your practice. Allow yourself to move with curiosity and compassion, listening to what your body needs at this moment. Trust that whatever unfolds is exactly what you need today. Embrace the journey, wherever it takes you, with a sense of openness and acceptance. In this way, your practice becomes less about achieving and more about experiencing. It's about being fully present, allowing each breath and movement to be a reflection of where you are right now—without judgment, without comparison, simply with acceptance.

Closing: As we close our practice, take a moment to let go of any remaining expectations you may have held for today. Honor the experience you had whatever it may have been knowing that it was exactly what you needed in this moment.

Opening: "Breathe in Possibility: Embracing New Beginnings with Each Breath"

As we begin our practice, take a moment to reflect on this simple yet profound mantra. With each inhale, imagine drawing in the energy of new possibilities, filling yourself with the potential of the future. Feel the breath expanding your chest, creating space within your body and mind for fresh starts and new beginnings. Let this breath be a symbol of the open road ahead, filled with opportunities to grow, learn, and evolve. As you exhale, consciously release anything from the past that no longer serves your old patterns, lingering doubts, or unresolved emotions. Imagine letting go of the weight of yesterday, feeling it dissolve with each breath out. This release creates a sense of lightness and freedom, making room for what lies ahead. In this way, your breath becomes a powerful tool for transformation. With every inhale, you invite the future full of hope, dreams, and aspirations. With every exhale, you let go of the past allowing it to rest, acknowledging it without holding on. This practice of consciously breathing in the future and releasing the past helps you to stay rooted in the present moment. It reminds you that while the past has shaped you, it does not define you, and that the future is a canvas waiting to be painted with your intentions. As we move through our practice today, carry this mantra with you. Use it as a gentle reminder to embrace change, welcome growth, and remain open to the endless possibilities that lie ahead. Allow your breath to guide you, creating space within yourself for new beginnings, both on and off the mat.

Closing: As we close our practice, return to that simple yet profound mantra we began with the inhale as an invitation for new possibilities, and the exhale as a release of what no longer serves you. Feel the energy of your breath, filling you with the potential of all that lies ahead, and creating space for growth and transformation. Recognize how each inhale expands your chest and mind, making room for fresh starts and new beginnings. And each exhale, a conscious release of any old patterns, doubts, or emotions that no longer serve you allowing you to feel lighter and more at ease. As you step off your mat, remember that this practice is not just about movement, but about staying rooted in the present, embracing the unfolding future with hope, and gently letting go of the past. Carry this intention with you: breathe in your dreams and aspirations; breathe out the weight of yesterday. Trust in your journey, and let your breath be your guide as you embrace the open road ahead.

Opening: "Come as You Are: Embracing Every Part of Yourself on the Mat"

This simple yet powerful invitation reminds us that yoga is a practice for everyone, in every state of being. When you step onto your mat, there's no need to leave parts of yourself at the door. Whether you're feeling strong and energized or tired and heavy-hearted, everything you bring to the mat is valid and welcome.

Arrive on your mat with an open heart and mind. This means letting go of any judgments or expectations about how your practice should look today. Some days, your body may feel flexible and capable, while on others, it might feel tight or fatigued. Your mind might be calm and focused, or it could be restless and distracted. Whatever you're experiencing, allow yourself to meet it with compassion. Yoga isn't about perfect poses or flawless sequences it's about being present with yourself exactly as you are. When you embrace all that you bring to the mat, you honor your true self. You acknowledge that your practice is a reflection of your current state, not a measure of your worth or ability.

Little Nugget: (longer hold) "Come as you are" also encourages you to let go of comparison. It's easy to look around the room and see others in their practice, but your journey is uniquely yours. By embracing your own experience, you create a space where you can explore, grow, and heal at your own pace. As you move through your practice, let this phrase remind you to be gentle with yourself. If a pose feels challenging today, honor that feeling. If you're carrying emotional weight, allow yourself to feel it without pushing it away. Your practice is a safe space to explore your physical, mental, and emotional landscape. When you come as you are, you give yourself permission to be authentic, vulnerable, and real. This is where true growth happens not by striving to be something else, but by fully embracing who you are in this moment. And in doing so, you open the door to deeper self-acceptance and a richer, more meaningful practice.

Closing: As we close our practice today, remember the invitation to 'come as you are.' You've taken the time to honor your own journey, moving through each pose and each breath at your own pace, without comparison or judgment. Take a moment to acknowledge the space you've created space for growth, healing, and self-acceptance. Reflect on how you embrace your challenges, listen to your body, and allow your emotions to simply be, without needing to change or fix them. By coming to your mat as you are authentic, vulnerable, and real you've allowed yourself to experience true growth, rooted not in striving, but in being. Carry this openness with you beyond your practice, knowing that by embracing who you are in each moment, you open the door to deeper self-love and acceptance.

Opening: "A Fresh Start: Embracing the Power to Begin Again"

Every time we step onto our mat, we have a chance to begin anew. Yoga invites us to start fresh with each practice, meeting ourselves exactly as we are free of judgment or comparison. Today's practice is a new experience, a new journey, an opportunity to tune in to your body and honor its needs. Coming to the mat with the body you have today means practicing mindfulness and self-compassion. It's about noticing how your body feels right now, letting go of past achievements and releasing any expectations for the future. Each practice reflects where you are in this moment, both physically and mentally. By letting go of yesterday's expectations, you create space for true growth and transformation. You become fully present, moving with intention and responding to your body's cues with kindness and respect. This approach not only deepens your connection to your practice but also nurtures a healthier, more loving relationship with your body.

Little Nugget: Feel the natural rise and fall of your breath, like a gentle rhythm connecting you to your inner self.

Closing: As we close our practice, take a moment to honor this fresh start you've created for yourself today. By letting go of past expectations and simply being present, you allowed yourself to connect deeply with your body and your breath. Remember that every time you come to your mat, you have this opportunity to begin again, to listen, to grow, and to honor yourself exactly as you are. Carry this sense of mindfulness and self-compassion with you beyond the mat, knowing that each moment is a chance to start anew. Take one final breath in, filling yourself with gratitude and openness, and a slow, gentle breath out, letting go of anything that no longer serves you.

Opening: "Grounded Presence: Cultivating Awareness in the Here and Now"

Take a moment to settle into this space. Leave behind the

busyness of the day, the distractions of the mind. Feel the mat beneath you, the earth supporting you. With every breath, let yourself arrive more fully in this present moment. This is your time, your space for connection, reflection, and renewal.

Closing: As we close our practice, return to the sense of presence you cultivated at the beginning arriving fully on your mat, in this space, and in this moment. Notice how, throughout our time together, you've allowed yourself to let go of the busyness of the day and the distractions of the mind, connecting deeply to the support beneath you and the breath within you. Remember that this sense of arrival isn't limited to your practice it's something you can carry with you into your life. Each moment is an invitation to pause, to connect, and to renew. As you step off your mat, take with you that sense of groundedness and peace, knowing that you can always return to it, simply by arriving fully in the present. Take a deep breath in, acknowledging this time you've given to yourself, and exhale softly, letting it ground you in the here and now.

Opening: "Flow with Change: Embracing Transformation On and Off the Mat"

As we step onto the mat, remember that change is constant, both in life and in our practice. Today, we embrace change whether it's the changing seasons, shifting emotions, or new challenges. Instead of resisting, let's flow with the change and trust where it takes us.

Closing: As we close our practice, remember to embrace the flow of change, both on and off the mat. Trust in the journey, knowing that every shift and challenge is guiding you to grow. When we move with change instead of resisting it, we find new strength, new possibilities, and a deeper sense of peace. Let go, flow, and trust the path that unfolds.

Seasonal Inspirations:

Opening: "Rooted in Nature: An Earth Day Practice for Grounding and Connection"

Welcome to your practice today. As we gather on our mats, let's take a moment to honor Earth Day. A day to celebrate the planet we all call home and reflect on our connection to it. The Earth supports us, grounds us, and nourishes us in every way. Just as the earth is steady and resilient, we can use this practice to find our own sense of grounding and connection.

As you settle into your space, feel the mat beneath you, knowing that it's an extension of the earth holding you up. Notice the way your body connects to the ground, and let each inhale fill you with a sense of stability and support. And with each exhale, imagine sending gratitude down into the earth, honoring all that it provides.

Today, let your practice be a way to root yourself in the present moment, finding strength in your foundation and allowing that connection to flow through you. Breathe in a sense of appreciation for the earth, and breathe out a commitment to protect, nurture, and honor this incredible home we share.

Closing: As we close our practice today, take a moment to reflect on the grounding energy you've cultivated and the deep connection you've felt with the earth. Just as the earth supports and nourishes us, may you carry that sense of stability and gratitude with you as you step off your mat. Remember that every breath you take is a gift from the earth, and each exhale is a way to give back. Let this practice inspire you to move through your day with care and respect for the world around you, grounded in the knowledge that we are all connected to this beautiful planet. Take one last deep breath in, drawing in the strength and support of the earth, and a gentle breath out, sending love and gratitude back down. May you walk forward rooted, centered, and ready to honor our shared home.

Opening: Honoring Memorial Day with Presence and Gratitude

Welcome to your practice today. As we gather on our mats, let's take a moment to honor Memorial Day a day of remembrance for those who have served and sacrificed. Today is not only about reflection but also about gratitude for the freedoms we enjoy and the lives we live. Start by finding a comfortable seat or lying down, gently closing your eyes. Take a deep breath in, filling your lungs with gratitude, and then exhale, letting go of any distractions or tension. Let's allow this practice to be a space of honoring and remembering, as well as a time to cultivate peace and presence within ourselves. As you move through today's practice, consider dedicating each breath and each movement to those who have given selflessly. Let this be a time to connect with your heart, to reflect on the deeper values of service, courage, and love for others.

Together, let's create space for gratitude for those who have served, for the life we live today, and for our own ability to show up with intention, compassion, and strength. Let's begin our practice, breathing in remembrance and breathing out gratitude.

Closing: As we come to the close of our practice, take a moment to find stillness and return to your breath. Place one hand on your heart and the other on your belly, feeling the rhythm of your breath as it rises and falls. Allow this connection to ground you in gratitude and remembrance. Take a deep breath in, filling yourself with appreciation for those who have served and for all the freedoms we hold dear. With your exhale, let go of anything that doesn't serve you, releasing any tension, stress, or distractions that may have surfaced. Let's take one more breath together, honoring the strength, courage, and selflessness of those we remember today. In your own way, silently offer a thought, a prayer, or a feeling of thanks for those who have sacrificed, as well as for your own ability to live with intention and purpose. Bow your head gently, acknowledging the light within you, the light in those around you, and the light in those we honor today.

Opening: "Shine Bright: Embracing Light and Expansion on the Summer Solstice"

Welcome to your practice today. As we gather together on this Summer Solstice, we honor the longest day of the year, a time of light, energy, and abundance. The sun is at its peak, filling our days with warmth and brightening all that it touches. Today, we celebrate this light not just the light around us but also the light within us. The Summer Solstice is a moment of expansion, growth, and fullness. Just as the sun stretches to its highest point in the sky, we are invited to open our hearts, reach for our fullest potential, and soak in all the energy that surrounds us. As you settle onto your mat, feel the warmth within your body, the energy flowing through your breath, and the openness of your heart. Let's take a moment to set an intention to honor this light both inside and out. As you breathe in, imagine drawing in the sun's warmth and radiance, allowing it to fill you with vitality and joy. And as you breathe out, release any heaviness or tension, making space for lightness and expansion.

Today, let your practice be a celebration of life, energy, and the beauty of being fully present. Embrace the light of the sun, the light within you, and let's move with gratitude for all that this season brings.

Closing: As we close our practice today, take a moment to honor the light you've cultivated the warmth, energy, and expansion that the Summer Solstice inspires. Feel the brightness within you, knowing that the same sun that lights the world shines within your own heart. Carry this sense of joy, openness, and vitality with you, letting the energy of this day infuse all that you do. Remember that just as the sun reaches its peak, you, too, have the power to stand fully in your light and share it with the world. Take one final, deep breath in, drawing in the sun's warmth and strength, and a slow, gentle breath out, releasing anything that no longer serves you, making space for the light to keep growing. May you walk forward from your mat today feeling radiant, energized, and ready to embrace the fullness of life.

Opening: Honoring Labor Day with a Practice of Rest and Renewal

Welcome to your practice today. As we gather on this Labor Day, let's take a moment to honor the spirit of the day a celebration of hard work, dedication, and the contributions of all those who labor, both seen and unseen. Today is also a reminder of the importance of rest and renewal, and an opportunity to pause, reflect, and honor your own efforts and the work you put into your life each day.

Take a comfortable seat or lie down, close your eyes, and begin to connect with your breath. Breathe in deeply, feeling the fullness of your breath filling your lungs, and as you exhale, let go of the demands and pressures of daily life. Let this time on your mat be a space to honor your own efforts and to find balance between work and rest, effort and ease. As you move through today's practice, let it be a time to celebrate all that you do. Embrace this moment to release any stress or tension that may have accumulated from your responsibilities. Acknowledge all the ways you show up in the world and all the hard work you've done not just in your job, but also in nurturing relationships, taking care of yourself, and contributing to your community.

Closing: As we close our practice, take a few moments to find stillness once more, allowing your breath to slow down and settle. Place one hand on your heart and the other on your belly, and feel the gentle rise and fall of your breath. Acknowledge the balance of effort and ease that you brought to your mat today. Take a deep breath in, honoring all the work you do in your life your strength, your dedication, and your commitment. And as you exhale, let go of any lingering tension, stress, or self-judgment, giving yourself permission to rest and renew. Labor Day is a reminder to honor not only your work but also the need for rest and self-care. As you step off your mat, carry with you this sense of balance and gratitude for all that you do and for the moments you allow yourself to simply be. Take one last deep breath in together, filling up with appreciation, and exhale, letting go with a sense of lightness and peace.

Opening:"Finding Equilibrium: A Fall Equinox Practice of Balance and Release"

Welcome to your practice today. As we gather on our mats, we honor the Fall Equinox a time when day and night are in perfect balance. This moment of equal light and darkness invites us to reflect on balance in our own lives. Just as nature begins to shift, we too can explore the balance between effort and ease, activity and rest, and holding on and letting go. The Equinox also marks the beginning of fall, a season of release and transformation. Just as the trees begin to shed their leaves, we're invited to let go of what no longer serves us, creating space for growth and renewal. Throughout our practice today, let's explore this balance within ourselves, finding moments to hold steady and moments to let go, allowing ourselves to flow with the natural rhythm of change. As you settle onto your mat, take a deep breath in, feeling the balance of this moment, and a long breath out, releasing anything that feels heavy. Let this practice be a celebration of balance, grounding, and gentle release.

Closing: As we close our practice today, take a moment to reflect on the balance you've cultivated—between effort and ease, between holding on and letting go. Just as the Fall Equinox marks the point of equal light and darkness, may you carry a sense of harmony within yourself as you move off the mat and into your life. Remember the invitation of this season—to let go of what no longer serves you, just as the trees release their leaves. Trust that in letting go, you create space for something new to grow. Take a deep breath in, honoring this balance and this season of transformation, and a long, gentle breath out, releasing anything you wish to leave behind.

Opening Theme: Cultivating Self-Love and Connection – A Valentine's Day Practice

Welcome to your practice today. As we gather on this Valentine's Day, let's take a moment to explore the deeper meaning of love the kind that starts within. While this day is often focused on expressing love to others, it's also a beautiful opportunity to connect with and honor the love we have for ourselves. Valentine's Day is a reminder to open our hearts to ourselves, to those around us, and to life. As you settle onto your mat, place one hand on your heart and the other on your belly. Take a deep breath in, feeling the rise and fall of your body, and let your exhale soften into a feeling of warmth and compassion. Let this practice be a gift to yourself a time to nurture, to listen, and to embrace all parts of who you are. With every breath, invite in a sense of kindness, acceptance, and love. Let's move through this practice today with an open heart, celebrating the love we have to give and receive, both on and off the mat.

Closing: As we close our practice today, take a moment to honor the love and compassion you've cultivated on your mat. Feel the gentle rhythm of your breath, the warmth in your heart, and the sense of connection you've created within yourself. Remember that Valentine's Day is not just about showing love to others, but also about nurturing and embracing the love you hold for yourself. Carry this self-love and acceptance with you as you step off your mat, letting it guide your actions and interactions. Let your breath continue to soften and open your heart, allowing you to give and receive love freely, without judgment, and with a sense of deep gratitude. Take one final breath in, filling yourself with warmth, kindness, and love, and a long, slow exhale, releasing into a state of peace and openness.

Opening: Celebrating Connection on International Yoga Day

Welcome to your practice, and happy International Yoga Day! Today, we join millions of people around the world to celebrate the unifying power of yoga. This day is a beautiful reminder that yoga is so much more than poses on a mat it's a practice that connects body, mind, and spirit, and unites communities across the globe. Take a moment to find a comfortable seat, close your eyes, and tune into your breath. With each inhale, feel yourself becoming more grounded and centered. With each exhale, imagine releasing anything that may be holding you back from fully embracing this moment. Let this breath connect you not just to yourself but to the wider yoga community, each breath a thread that weaves us all together. Today's practice is about honoring what yoga means to you, whether it's a journey of self-discovery, healing, strength, or balance. It's also a day to celebrate the unity and connection that yoga fosters in all of us. As we move together, know that you're part of something much bigger a shared experience that transcends boundaries and brings light, love, and awareness to the world. Let's breathe in connection, breathe out gratitude, and flow in celebration of this beautiful practice. Let's begin.

Closing: As we come to the close of our practice, take a few moments to return to your breath and find stillness. Gently close your eyes, place one hand on your heart, and the other on your belly, feeling the breath as it rises and falls. Reflect on this shared moment of unity how yoga has connected us not only to ourselves but also to each other and to the wider world. Today, we celebrated yoga's ability to bring balance, peace, and joy into our lives, and we honored our place in the global yoga community. Take a deep breath in, breathing in connection and love, and as you exhale, let go of anything that doesn't serve you, sending gratitude to yourself for showing up, and to the millions of others who join you in this practice today. As you step off your mat, carry this feeling of unity, compassion, and light with you. Let your practice ripple outward, bringing the peace you found here to everything you touch.

Opening: Embracing the Energy of the Full Moon

Welcome to your practice on this full moon night a time of heightened energy, illumination, and reflection. The full moon symbolizes completion, fullness, and release. Just as the moon shines brightly, revealing everything in its light, tonight we have an opportunity to turn inward and reflect on what has come to completion in our own lives. The full moon is a time to celebrate all that you've accomplished and to let go of what you've outgrown. It's a moment to release any old habits, thoughts, or energies that no longer serve you, making space for new intentions to grow. Throughout our practice, let the moon's energy inspire you to open up, to shine brightly, and to release what you no longer need. As you settle onto your mat, take a deep breath in, welcoming the moon's illuminating energy into your body, and a deep breath out, letting go of any heaviness or resistance. Let's move together under this full moon with clarity, intention, and the freedom to embrace change.

Closing: As we close our practice under the full moon's energy, take a moment to honor all that has come to the surface. Just as the full moon illuminates the night, bringing clarity and reflection, may this practice have brought light to any parts of yourself ready to be seen, celebrated, or released. Reflect on what you are ready to let go of old habits, thoughts, or energies and know that by releasing them, you create space for new possibilities to arise. Just as the moon eventually begins to wane, let go with grace, knowing that change is a natural rhythm of life. Take one last deep breath in, drawing in the moon's energy and clarity, and a long breath out, letting go of anything that no longer serves you. May you move forward with lightness, openness, and the peace of knowing you are always evolving.

Opening: A Gratitude-Filled Practice for Thanksgiving
 Tip: Have each student write what they are grateful for on a piece of paper and have them leave it at the top of their mat so that it serves as a reminder throughout practice.

Welcome, everyone. As we gather on our mats today, let's take a moment to connect with the essence of Thanksgiving gratitude. This season is a beautiful opportunity to pause, reflect, and appreciate all the blessings in our lives, both big and small. Start by settling into a comfortable seat or lying down, closing your eyes, and tuning into your breath. With each inhale, imagine breathing in appreciation and thankfulness. With each exhale, let go of any tension or distractions, allowing yourself to be fully present. As you move through your practice today, consider this an invitation to cultivate gratitude not just for the joys, but also for the challenges that have helped you grow, the connections that support you, and the body that carries you through each day. This practice is a time to honor all the things we often take for granted the breath that fills our lungs, the earth beneath us, and the ability to move, stretch, and feel. Let this be a practice of giving thanks for exactly where you are, who you are, and all that you are capable of becoming. Closing: As we come to the end of our practice, take a few moments to settle back into stillness. Allow your breath to slow down, and let yourself rest in the gratitude we've cultivated today. Place one hand on your heart and the other on your belly, feeling the warmth of your own touch. Take a deep breath in, and with your exhale, let a wave of appreciation flow through your body gratitude for your practice, for your breath, for showing up on your mat, and for all that is unfolding in your life. Let the feelings of thanks and love radiate from your heart, imagining them spreading not just through your body but outward into the world. Remember that gratitude is a practice we can return to at any moment, on and off the mat, to find peace, perspective, and connection.

Take one more deep breath in, filling up with all that you are thankful for, and as you exhale, release any lingering tension or thoughts. With a bow of your head, acknowledge the light within yourself and the light in others. Thank you for sharing this space and this practice.

Opening: Christmas Eve

May this practice be a moment of peace, joy, and gratitude amidst the season's busyness. Just as we celebrate the light and love of Christmas, let us also honor the light within ourselves. As we move and breathe today, may we cultivate a sense of warmth, connection, and generosity not just to others, but to ourselves as well. Let your mat be a place of stillness and reflection, where you can unwrap the gift of being present and whole.

Closing: As we close our practice, carry with you the peace, joy, and gratitude that you cultivated on your mat today. Let this sense of warmth and connection fill your heart and guide you through the rest of the season. Remember that just as we celebrate the light of Christmas, you also hold a bright, beautiful light within you one that you can share with others and nurture within yourself. Take one final deep breath in, filling up with that love and warmth, and a slow, gentle breath out, releasing any stress or tension. May you leave this space feeling present, whole, and full of the spirit of the season.

Opening: "A Heartfelt Celebration – A Christmas Day Practice"

Welcome, and Merry Christmas! Today is a day of warmth, connection, and giving, and as we gather on our mats, we take a moment to honor the spirit of the season. Christmas is a time to celebrate love, joy, and gratitude not just for the gifts we receive but for the gifts we carry within ourselves and share with others. As you settle in, close your eyes and take a deep breath in, feeling the lightness of the holiday fill your heart. Breathe in the joy, peace, and love of this day. And as you exhale, let go of any stress or busyness, allowing yourself to be fully present in this moment. Let your practice today be an act of self-care, a gift to yourself to move with intention, to breathe deeply, and to connect with the warmth and comfort of the season. May this time on your mat be a space of grounding, gratitude, and a reminder that the greatest gift you can give is your presence to yourself, to those you love, and to this moment. Let's move, breathe, and celebrate the beauty of Christmas together.

Closing: As we close our practice today, take a moment to reflect on the joy, peace, and love that fill this Christmas day. Let the warmth and light you've cultivated within radiate outward, connecting you to the spirit of the season and to all those you hold dear. Remember that this practice was a gift to yourself a time to pause, breathe, and find presence amidst the festivities. Carry this sense of gratitude and connection with you as you continue your day, knowing that the love and joy you nurture within are the most precious gifts you have to share. Take one final deep breath in, filling your heart with the spirit of Christmas, and a slow, gentle breath out, letting that peace settle into every part of your being.

Opening: "New Years Eve"

As we step onto our mats on this New Year's Eve, let each breath be a reflection of both release and renewal. Inhale the lessons and growth of the past year, and exhale to let go of anything you wish to leave behind. May this practice be a bridge between who you've been and who you're becoming an opportunity to find peace with the past and embrace the endless possibilities of the year to come.

Closing: As we close our practice and prepare to welcome the new year, take a moment to honor this space you've created for reflection, release, and renewal. Let go of any heaviness or tension, and breathe in the hope and possibility that the new year brings.

Carry forward the lessons, joys, and growth of the past year, and leave behind what no longer serves you. Trust in the journey ahead and remember that each moment is a chance to begin again. Take one final deep breath in, filling yourself with gratitude and intention, and a slow, cleansing breath out, releasing fully into the promise of a fresh start.

Opening: "A Fresh Start – A New Year's Day Practice"

Welcome to a brand new year and a brand new practice. Today, as we step onto our mats, we celebrate fresh beginnings a chance to reset, renew, and open ourselves up to the possibilities of the year ahead. New Year's Day is a time to reflect on what you wish to create, release, and welcome into your life. As you settle in, close your eyes and take a deep breath in, feeling the expansiveness of this moment a moment of pure potential. Let your breath symbolize a fresh start, an invitation to step into this new year with intention and an open heart. With every inhale, breathe in hope, clarity, and purpose. With every exhale, let go of any lingering doubts, stress, or expectations that may hold you back. Today, let your practice be a dedication to yourself, a celebration of how far you've come, and a commitment to the journey ahead. Remember, each breath is a new beginning, and each movement is a chance to plant seeds for the future. Let's embrace this moment, this new year, and all the beauty it holds.

Closing: As we close our practice on this New Year's Day, take a moment to honor the fresh start you've created both on your mat and in your life. Feel the energy of renewal within you, and remember that each breath is a new opportunity to grow, transform, and step into the person you wish to become. Reflect on the intentions you've set and carry them forward with you, knowing that this practice is not just a moment but a journey one that continues far beyond the mat. With gratitude for the past and excitement for the future, may you walk into this new year with clarity, purpose, and an open heart. Take one last deep breath in, inviting in all the possibilities of the year ahead, and a slow, gentle breath out, releasing into the peace of this new beginning.

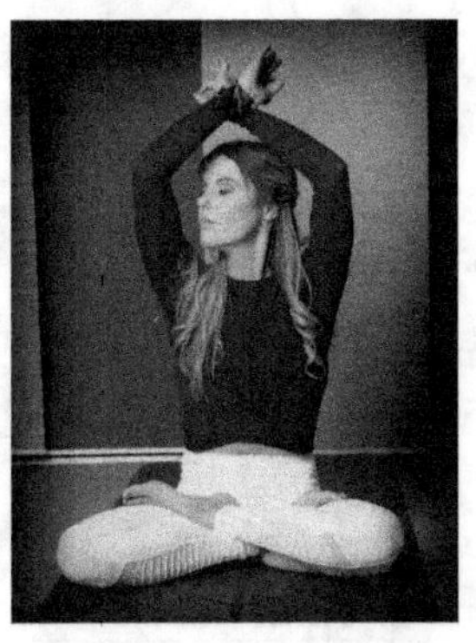

About the Author

Alyson has over 15 years of experience teaching yoga to students, and for more than a decade, she has been guiding new teachers through transformative teacher trainings. With a passion for helping others find their authentic voice, Alyson provides "done-for-you" programs designed to build confidence and empower yoga teachers on their journey. As a Reiki healer and spiritual coach, she brings a deep understanding of energy work and personal growth to her teachings, supporting her students in cultivating a strong mind-body connection and living more balanced, empowered lives.

Ready to transform your yoga teaching journey? Whether you're looking to build confidence, find your authentic voice, or deepen your understanding of energy work, Alyson's 'done-for-you' programs offer the tools and support you need. Step into your power as a teacher, connect deeply with yourself and your students, and live a more balanced, empowered life. Reach out to Alyson email: youryogabizz@gmail.com or register for her newsletter below.

You can connect with me on:
- 🌐 https://www.beachbumyogafl.com/your-yoga-bizz
- 🔗 https://www.instagram.com/youryogabizz

Subscribe to my newsletter:
- ✉ https://alysonjune.myflodesk.com/edchb6t3zs

www.ingramcontent.com/pod-product-compliance
Lightning Source LLC
Chambersburg PA
CBHW051700250726
48653CB00007B/2766